PILATES FOR THERAPY

A Comprehensive Guide To Pain Relief,
Rehabilitation, And Strength Building
Through Targeted Exercises

DR. MELISSA STOTLER

Copyright © 2023 by Dr. Melissa Stotler

All rights reserved. Except for brief quotations embodied in critical reviews and certain other noncommercial uses permitted by copyright law, no part of this publication may be reproduced, distributed, or transmitted in any form or by any means, Including photocopying, recording, or other electronic or mechanical methods, without the prior written permission of the publisher.

Disclaimer:

The data in this book, "Acupuncture Therapy Simplified," is solely meant to be informative and instructional.

This book is not intended to replace expert medical advice, diagnosis, or care. No medical, health, or other professional services are offered by the author, publisher, or any affiliated parties

Individual outcomes may differ in the practice of these therapies, which entail a variety of approaches and methodologies.

A one-on-one session with a trained or certified healthcare professional is still preferable. It is best to consult a trained healthcare provider before making any decisions regarding your health.

The author of this book is not affiliated with any specific website, product, or organization related to any of these therapies.

All reasonable measures have been taken by the author and publisher to guarantee the authenticity and dependability of the material contained in this book.

Contents

CHAPTER ONE 10
  UNDERSTANDING PILATES FUNDAMENTALS 10
    Importance Of Alignment And Posture 13
    Basic Anatomy For Pilates Practitioners 14
    Common Beginner Mistakes And How To Avoid Them 16
    Using Momentum 17

CHAPTER TWO 19
  BREATHING TECHNIQUES IN PILATES 19
    The Role Of Breath In Pilates 19
    Diaphragmatic Breathing 20
    Lateral Thoracic Breathing 21
    Incorporating Breath With Movement 22
    Breathing Exercises For Practice 23

CHAPTER THREE 25
  CORE STRENGTH AND STABILITY 25
    Importance Of Core Muscles In Pilates 25
    Exercises To Strengthen The Core 26
    Modifications For Different Fitness Levels 28
    Using Props To Enhance Core Workouts 29
    Progressing Core Exercises Over Time 31

CHAPTER FOUR 33
  PILATES MAT EXERCISES 33
    Essential Mat Exercises For Beginners 33
    Progressions To Intermediate And Advanced Mat Exercises 35

Incorporating Small Props: Bands, Balls, And Rings 37

Creating A Balanced Mat Routine 38

Tips For Practicing Mat Pilates At Home 40

CHAPTER FIVE 42

PILATES REFORMER EXERCISES 42

Basic Reformer Exercises And Their Benefits 43

Adjusting The Reformer For Different Body Types 45

Safety And Maintenance Of The Reformer 47

Integrating Reformer Workouts Into Your Routine 49

CHAPTER SIX 52

PILATES FOR SPECIFIC CONDITIONS 52

Pilates For Back Pain Relief 52

Pilates For Joint Health And Mobility 53

Pilates For Post-Surgery Recovery 55

Modifications For Chronic Conditions 56

Real-Life Success Stories And Testimonials 57

CHAPTER SEVEN 59

ADVANCED PILATES TECHNIQUES 59

Transitioning From Beginner To Advanced Exercises 59

Challenging The Body With Complex Movements 60

Using Advanced Equipment: Cadillac, Chair, And Barrel 61

Combining Pilates With Other Fitness Routines 62

Preventing Injuries During Advanced Practice 63

CHAPTER EIGHT 65

CREATING A PERSONALIZED PILATES PROGRAM 65

    Assessing Individual Needs And Goals 65

    Designing A Balanced Weekly Pilates Schedule 66

    Mixing Mat And Equipment Workouts 67

    Adapting Routines For Progress And Variety 68

    Evaluating And Adjusting Your Program Over Time 69

CHAPTER NINE 70

    COMMON CONCERNS AND FAQS 70

    Addressing Common Fears And Misconceptions 70

    Dealing With Soreness And Fatigue 71

    Finding The Right Balance Between Effort And Rest 72

    Answers to Frequently Asked Questions About Pilates 73

    Tips For Staying Committed And Enjoying Your Practice 75

ABOUT THIS BOOK

"Pilates for Therapy" delves deeply into the principles and practices of Pilates, highlighting its therapeutic benefits. This book begins by laying a solid foundation with a comprehensive understanding of Pilates fundamentals. It explores the six core principles—Concentration, Control, Centering, Flow, Precision, and Breathing—essential for mastering Pilates. The importance of alignment and posture is emphasized, offering readers insights into basic anatomy and common terminology. The book also addresses common beginner mistakes, guiding how to avoid them for a safe and effective practice.

The role of breathing in Pilates is meticulously detailed, with a focus on diaphragmatic and lateral thoracic breathing. Readers will learn how to incorporate breath with movement, enhancing the efficiency and effectiveness of their workouts. Practical breathing exercises are included to help practitioners develop proper breathing techniques integral to Pilates.

Core strength and stability are central themes, highlighting the importance of core muscles in Pilates practice. The book presents various exercises to strengthen the core, with modifications for different fitness levels. It also discusses the use of props to enhance core workouts and offers strategies for progressing these exercises over time, ensuring continuous improvement and challenge.

Pilates mat exercises form a crucial part of this guide, featuring essential exercises for beginners and progressions to more advanced levels. The integration of small props such as bands, balls, and rings adds variety and effectiveness to routines. Tips for practicing mat Pilates at home provide readers with the tools to create balanced, effective workouts in their own space.

The introduction to Pilates Reformer exercises opens up new dimensions of the practice. This section covers basic Reformer exercises, their benefits, and how to adjust the Reformer for different body types. Safety and maintenance tips ensure that readers can use this equipment effectively and confidently integrate Reformer workouts into their routines.

Addressing specific conditions, the book explores how Pilates can aid in back pain relief, joint health, and post-surgery recovery. Modifications for chronic conditions make Pilates accessible to a wider audience, while real-life success stories and testimonials offer inspiration and encouragement.

For those ready to advance their practice, the book guides transitioning to advanced exercises and using equipment like the Cadillac, Chair, and Barrel. It emphasizes the importance of preventing injuries and combining Pilates with other fitness routines for a well-rounded approach.

Creating a personalized Pilates program is made easy with advice on assessing individual needs and goals, designing a balanced schedule, and mixing mat and equipment workouts. The book offers strategies for adapting routines over time to maintain progress and variety, ensuring long-term commitment and enjoyment.

Common concerns and FAQs are addressed, dispelling fears and misconceptions.

Practical advice on dealing with soreness, finding the right balance between effort and rest, and tips for staying committed enrich the journey into the world of Pilates. This comprehensive guide is designed to make Pilates accessible, enjoyable, and beneficial for everyone, regardless of their fitness level or specific needs.

CHAPTER ONE

UNDERSTANDING PILATES FUNDAMENTALS

Pilates is a form of exercise that emphasizes the balanced development of the body through core strength, flexibility, and awareness to support efficient, graceful movement. Developed by Joseph Pilates in the early 20th century, this method is now widely recognized for its ability to enhance physical and mental well-being.

The Six Principles of Pilates: Concentration, Control, Centering, Flow, Precision, and Breathing

Concentration

Concentration is key in Pilates. Each movement requires full mental focus to ensure that exercises are performed correctly and effectively. By concentrating on each exercise, you improve your form, maximize results, and reduce the risk of injury.

Control

Pilates is sometimes called "Contrology," as it emphasizes controlling every part of your body. This control helps in performing exercises with accuracy, engaging the appropriate muscles, and maintaining proper form. Movements should be deliberate, avoiding any sloppy or uncontrolled actions.

Centering

All Pilates exercises stem from the core, also known as the "powerhouse." This area includes your abdomen, lower back, hips, and buttocks. Strengthening the core is fundamental in Pilates as it provides stability and support for the entire body.

Flow

Flow, or the smooth transition between movements, is crucial in Pilates. Exercises are performed in a fluid, graceful manner, without jerky or abrupt movements. This continuous flow enhances the coordination and balance of the body.

Precision

Precision in Pilates ensures that each movement is executed with meticulous attention to detail. Proper alignment and muscle engagement are crucial for achieving the desired outcomes of each exercise. Practicing precision leads to better results and helps in correcting imbalances in the body.

Breathing

Breathing is integral to Pilates. Proper breathing techniques help oxygenate the muscles, increase relaxation, and support effective muscle engagement.

Typically, Pilates incorporates deep, diaphragmatic breathing, coordinating breath with movement to enhance performance and concentration.

Importance Of Alignment And Posture

Alignment and posture are central to the effectiveness of Pilates exercises. Proper alignment ensures that the body is in its optimal position, reducing the risk of injury and maximizing the efficiency of each movement.

Good posture supports the spine and allows for better breathing and overall function. In Pilates, emphasis is placed on maintaining a neutral spine, which preserves the natural curves of the back.

Practitioners are taught to be aware of their alignment throughout exercises, ensuring that the head, shoulders, and hips are in proper alignment. This awareness extends beyond the Pilates session, promoting better posture in daily activities.

Basic Anatomy For Pilates Practitioners

A fundamental understanding of anatomy is beneficial for Pilates practitioners. Knowing the basic structure of the body helps in identifying which muscles are being engaged and understanding the mechanics of each movement. Key anatomical concepts include:

The Core Muscles: Includes the transverse abdominis, rectus abdominis, obliques, and the muscles of the lower back and pelvic floor.

The Spine: Understanding the sections of the spine (cervical, thoracic, lumbar, sacral) and their natural curves is crucial.

Major Muscle Groups: Awareness of muscle groups such as the quadriceps, hamstrings, glutes, and shoulder girdle muscles aids in performing exercises correctly.

Joint Functionality: Knowing how joints move and the range of motion they should achieve helps in executing Pilates exercises safely and effectively.

Pilates Terminology

Pilates has its own set of terms that can seem confusing to beginners. Familiarizing yourself with these terms can enhance your practice:

Powerhouse: Refers to the core muscles.

Neutral Spine: Maintaining the natural curves of the spine.

Pelvic Floor: The muscles supporting the base of the pelvis.

Articulation: The action of moving one vertebra at a time.

C-Curve: A position where the spine forms a C-shape, engaging the core muscles.

Common Beginner Mistakes And How To Avoid Them

Incorrect Breathing

Many beginners forget to coordinate their breath with movement, leading to ineffective exercises. Focus on deep, diaphragmatic breathing, and match your breath to your movements.

Overarching the Back

Maintaining a neutral spine can be challenging for beginners, who often tend to overarch their back. Engage your core and focus on keeping your spine in a neutral position throughout the exercises.

Using Momentum

Beginners often use momentum instead of muscle control to perform movements. Slow down your exercises and concentrate on controlled, deliberate movements.

Ignoring Form

Form is crucial in Pilates, and ignoring it can lead to injury. Pay close attention to your alignment and muscle engagement. Use mirrors or seek guidance from a qualified instructor to ensure proper form.

Not Engaging the Core

Pilates exercises are centered around the core, but beginners sometimes fail to engage these muscles properly. Focus on drawing your navel towards your spine and maintaining this engagement throughout the exercises.

By understanding these fundamental principles and common pitfalls, beginners can enhance their Pilates practice, achieving better results and fostering a deeper connection with their bodies.

CHAPTER TWO

BREATHING TECHNIQUES IN PILATES

The Role Of Breath In Pilates

Breathing is a fundamental element in Pilates, playing a crucial role in enhancing the effectiveness of exercises and ensuring proper execution. In Pilates, breath control aids in centering the body, providing stability, and fostering a mind-body connection that enhances focus and precision.

Correct breathing techniques ensure that muscles receive adequate oxygen, promoting endurance and reducing fatigue.

Additionally, synchronized breathing and movement help maintain a steady rhythm, enabling smoother and more controlled transitions between exercises.

Diaphragmatic Breathing

Diaphragmatic breathing, also known as abdominal or belly breathing, is essential in Pilates for engaging the core and maintaining a strong, stable center.

This technique involves breathing deeply into the lower lungs by expanding the diaphragm.

When practicing diaphragmatic breathing, inhale deeply through the nose, allowing the abdomen to rise as the diaphragm moves downward.

Exhale slowly through the mouth, feeling the abdomen contract as the diaphragm moves back up.

This method not only improves oxygen flow but also activates the deep abdominal muscles, essential for core stability in Pilates exercises.

Lateral Thoracic Breathing

Lateral thoracic breathing, or rib cage breathing, emphasizes the expansion of the rib cage rather than the abdomen.

This technique is particularly beneficial in Pilates as it encourages the engagement of the intercostal muscles and enhances the flexibility and mobility of the thoracic spine.

To practice lateral thoracic breathing, inhale deeply through the nose, focusing on expanding the ribs outward and sideways. Exhale through the mouth, feeling the ribs contract and draw closer together.

This type of breathing supports the maintenance of a stable core while allowing for a greater range of motion in the upper body during Pilates exercises.

Incorporating Breath With Movement

Integrating breath with movement is a core principle of Pilates, ensuring that exercises are performed with maximum efficiency and control.

Each movement in Pilates is paired with a specific breathing pattern to enhance muscle engagement and movement precision.

For example, inhaling during the preparation phase of an exercise fills the lungs with oxygen, while exhaling during the exertion phase helps to stabilize the core and control the movement.

Practitioners are encouraged to synchronize their breath with their movements, allowing the breath to guide the rhythm and flow of each exercise, creating a harmonious and effective workout.

Breathing Exercises For Practice

To master the breathing techniques in Pilates, practitioners can incorporate specific breathing exercises into their routine. Here are a few exercises to enhance breathing control and efficiency:

Breathing Awareness: Lie on your back with your knees bent and feet flat on the floor. Place one hand on your abdomen and the other on your chest. Inhale deeply through your nose, feeling the abdomen rise, then exhale through your mouth, feeling the abdomen fall. Repeat, focusing on the movement of the diaphragm and the expansion of the lungs.

Rib Cage Expansion: Sit or stand with your spine elongated. Place your hands on your rib cage. Inhale deeply through your nose, feeling the ribs expand outward and sideways. Exhale through your mouth, allowing the ribs to contract. Practice this exercise to develop awareness and control of lateral thoracic breathing.

Coordinated Breathing: Begin in a seated or lying position. Inhale deeply through your nose, filling the lungs. Exhale through your mouth, engaging the core muscles. As you become comfortable, incorporate simple movements such as arm lifts or leg extensions, synchronizing the breath with the movement to practice integrating breath and motion.

By practicing these breathing techniques, Pilates practitioners can enhance their overall performance, ensuring that each exercise is executed with precision and control, and ultimately achieving the full benefits of their Pilates practice.

CHAPTER THREE

CORE STRENGTH AND STABILITY

Importance Of Core Muscles In Pilates

In Pilates, core strength is fundamental to achieving stability and effective movement. The core muscles, which include the abdominals, obliques, lower back, and pelvic floor, act as the body's central support system. These muscles stabilize the spine and pelvis, providing a solid foundation for every movement and exercise. A strong core enhances posture, balance, and coordination, making everyday activities and physical exercises more efficient and safer.

Core strength in Pilates is not just about achieving a flat stomach; it's about developing a deep, functional strength that supports the entire body. This internal strength allows for greater control during exercises and reduces the risk of injury by ensuring that the body is aligned and balanced. In essence, a well-developed core supports the body from the inside out, enabling smooth and coordinated movements.

Exercises To Strengthen The Core

Plank: Begin in a push-up position, with your weight supported on your hands and toes. Keep your body in a straight line from head to heels. Engage your core by pulling your belly button towards your spine. Hold this position for 20-60 seconds, depending on your fitness level.

The Hundred: Lie on your back with your legs lifted to a tabletop position. Curl your head and shoulders off the mat, reaching your arms long by your sides. Pump your arms up and down while taking five short breaths in and five short breaths out. Continue for 100 breaths, or as many as you can manage.

Single-Leg Stretch: Lie on your back with your head and shoulders lifted. Bring one knee towards your chest while extending the other leg out, hovering above the ground. Switch legs and repeat, pulling your knee towards your chest and extending the other leg. Perform 10-15 repetitions on each side.

Leg Circles: Lie on your back with one leg extended towards the ceiling. Keeping your hips stable, draw small circles with your raised leg. Perform 10-15 circles in each direction before switching legs.

Criss-Cross: Lie on your back with your hands behind your head and knees bent. Lift your head, shoulders, and legs into a tabletop position. Rotate your torso to bring one elbow towards the opposite knee while extending the other leg. Switch sides and repeat for 10-15 repetitions on each side.

Modifications For Different Fitness Levels

Not everyone will start at the same level of core strength, so it's important to modify exercises to accommodate individual fitness levels.

Beginners: For those new to Pilates or with lower core strength, starting with modified versions of core exercises can help build strength gradually. For example, in the Plank exercise, beginners can start by supporting their weight on their knees instead of their toes.

Intermediate: As core strength improves, standard versions of exercises can be introduced. For instance, performing the Plank with one leg lifted or with arm lifts can add an extra challenge.

Advanced: Advanced practitioners can incorporate variations like side planks, where the body is supported on one side, or adding resistance with weights or resistance bands during core exercises.

Using Props To Enhance Core Workouts

Props can be a valuable tool in Pilates for enhancing core workouts and adding variety to exercises.

Stability Ball: Placing your feet or hands on a stability ball during exercises like Planks or Roll-Ups can increase the challenge by adding instability. This forces the core muscles to work harder to maintain balance.

Foam Roller: Using a foam roller can enhance exercises by targeting deep core muscles. For example, performing the Plank with your shins resting on the foam roller can challenge your balance and engage your core more intensively.

Resistance Bands: Incorporating resistance bands can add extra resistance to exercises like the Hundred or Criss-Cross.

The bands can be anchored under your feet or hands to increase the intensity of your core workout.

Pilates Ring: The Pilates ring, also known as a magic circle, can be used to increase resistance in exercises like the Inner Thigh Squeeze or the Hundred. It helps engage specific muscle groups more effectively.

Progressing Core Exercises Over Time

As core strength develops, it's important to progressively challenge yourself to continue making improvements.

Increase Duration and Intensity: Gradually increase the time you hold each exercise, such as holding the Plank position for longer periods or performing more repetitions of The Hundred.

Add Variations: Introduce variations of exercises to keep your workouts challenging and engaging. For example, try different leg positions or combine core exercises for a more comprehensive routine.

Incorporate Advanced Techniques: As you build strength, you can incorporate advanced techniques such as using weighted vests or resistance bands to further enhance the effectiveness of your core workouts.

Monitor Progress: Regularly assess your progress by tracking improvements in your ability to perform exercises, your endurance, and overall core strength. Adjust your workout routine as needed to ensure continued growth and challenge.

By following these guidelines and incorporating these strategies, you can effectively develop and maintain core strength and stability through Pilates, leading to better overall fitness and well-being.

CHAPTER FOUR

PILATES MAT EXERCISES

Pilates mat exercises form the foundation of many Pilates routines and offer a versatile way to enhance strength, flexibility, and body awareness. These exercises are performed on the mat and can be modified to suit different skill levels, making them ideal for both beginners and advanced practitioners. By mastering the basic movements and progressively challenging yourself, you can achieve a well-rounded Pilates practice.

Essential Mat Exercises For Beginners

For those new to Pilates, starting with fundamental mat exercises is key to building a strong foundation. These exercises focus on improving core strength, flexibility, and overall body control.

The Pelvic Tilt: This exercise helps engage your lower abdominal muscles and improve lower back stability. Lie on your back with your knees bent and feet flat on the floor. Gently press your lower back into the mat by tilting your pelvis upward, then release. Repeat several times.

The Single Leg Stretch: This movement targets the abdominal muscles and helps with coordination. Lie on your back with your knees bent and lift your head, neck, and shoulders off the mat. Extend one leg out while pulling the other knee toward your chest. Alternate legs in a smooth, controlled motion.

The Cat-Cow Stretch: Ideal for improving spinal flexibility and mobility, this exercise involves moving between two positions. Start on your hands and knees, then arch your back and tuck your chin to your chest (Cat). Next, dip your back and lift your head and tailbone (Cow). Repeat this flow several times.

The Plank: This exercise strengthens the entire core while engaging the shoulders and back. Begin in a push-up position, with your body in a straight line from head to heels. Hold this position, making sure to keep your abs tight and your hips level.

Progressions To Intermediate And Advanced Mat Exercises

Once you are comfortable with the basic exercises, you can progress to more challenging movements that enhance strength and coordination.

The Roll-Up: This exercise works the entire core and improves spinal articulation. Lie on your back with your arms extended overhead. Slowly roll up to a seated position, reaching for your toes, and then roll back down. This exercise requires control and concentration.

The Teaser: A more advanced move, the Teaser strengthens the core and enhances balance. Begin by lying on your back with your legs extended and arms reaching toward the ceiling. Lift your legs and torso off the mat to create a V shape, then lower back down with control.

The Scissor Kick: This exercise targets the lower abs and hip flexors. Lie on your back with your legs extended and lift both legs to a 45-degree angle. Alternate crossing your legs over each other in a scissor-like motion, keeping your core engaged.

The Side Plank: This variation of the plank focuses on the obliques and side muscles. Lie on your side with your legs straight and prop yourself up on one elbow. Lift your hips to create a straight line from head to feet. Hold the position, then switch sides.

Incorporating Small Props: Bands, Balls, And Rings

Using small props in your Pilates mat routine can enhance your workout by adding variety and increasing resistance. Props such as resistance bands, stability balls, and Pilates rings are excellent tools for targeting specific muscle groups and improving overall strength.

Resistance Bands: These bands can be used to add resistance to exercises like the Leg Lift or the Glute Bridge. Secure the band around your legs or feet, and perform your exercises as usual. The added resistance helps increase muscle engagement and strength.

Stability Balls: A stability ball can be used to challenge your balance and core stability. Try exercises such as the Ball Pass, where you pass the ball between your hands and feet while lying on your back, or the Ball Roll-Out, where you roll the ball out in front of you while in a plank position.

Pilates Rings: The Pilates ring, or magic circle, is used to provide resistance and increase the intensity of exercises. Use it during exercises like the Inner Thigh Squeeze or the Chest Lift to engage and tone specific muscle groups more effectively.

Creating A Balanced Mat Routine

To maximize the benefits of your Pilates mat practice, it's important to create a balanced routine that targets all major muscle groups and addresses different aspects of fitness.

Warm-Up: Start with a gentle warm-up to prepare your muscles and joints for more intense work. Include exercises such as the Cat-Cow Stretch or the Roll Down to increase circulation and flexibility.

Core Work: Incorporate exercises that focus on core strength, such as the Plank or the Single Leg Stretch. A strong core supports overall stability and improves posture.

Lower Body: Include movements that target the lower body, such as the Leg Lift or the Glute Bridge. These exercises help build strength and endurance in the legs and hips.

Upper Body: Don't forget to include exercises that work the upper body, such as the Chest Lift or the Push-Up. These help to balance your workout and strengthen your arms and shoulders.

5. Flexibility and Cool Down: Finish with stretches and flexibility exercises to help your muscles recover and maintain range of motion. Include stretches like the Forward Fold or the Seated Twist.

Tips For Practicing Mat Pilates At Home

Practicing Pilates at home offers flexibility and convenience, but it's important to create an environment and routine that supports your practice.

Set Up a Dedicated Space: Create a comfortable, clutter-free area where you can practice Pilates regularly. Use a good-quality mat for cushioning and support.

Follow a Routine: Establish a regular practice schedule to build consistency. Whether it's a daily 15-minute session or longer workouts a few times a week, having a routine helps you stay committed.

Use Online Resources: Take advantage of online videos or classes to guide your practice. Many resources offer structured routines and tips for different skill levels.

Listen to Your Body: Pay attention to how your body feels during each exercise. Modify movements as needed and avoid pushing through pain.

Stay Hydrated and Rested: Proper hydration and rest are important for muscle recovery and overall well-being. Make sure to drink water before and after your practice and get enough rest to support your fitness goals.

CHAPTER FIVE

PILATES REFORMER EXERCISES

The Pilates Reformer is a versatile piece of equipment designed to enhance strength, flexibility, and overall fitness through controlled movements.

Its design includes a sliding carriage, adjustable springs, and various attachments like straps and bars.

By adjusting the resistance and using different accessories, the Reformer can be tailored to suit individual fitness levels and goals.

This makes it an ideal tool for both beginners and advanced practitioners seeking to improve their physical condition in a low-impact, controlled manner.

Basic Reformer Exercises And Their Benefits

Footwork

Footwork is a foundational Reformer exercise that targets the legs and lower body. Pressing the footbar with the feet while lying on the carriage, this exercise helps to strengthen the quadriceps, hamstrings, and calves. Footwork improves circulation and enhances lower body stability, which is crucial for overall movement efficiency.

The Hundred

This classic Pilates exercise involves lying on your back with the legs lifted and pumping the arms up and down. The Hundred is excellent for building core strength and endurance. It challenges the abdominal muscles and helps to improve breath control, which is essential for overall body stability and function.

Roll-Up

The Roll-Up exercise involves lying on the Reformer and slowly rolling up to a seated position before rolling back down. This exercise targets the abdominal muscles, improving spinal flexibility and strength. The Roll-Up is beneficial for enhancing posture and relieving back tension.

Leg Circles

While lying on the Reformer with one leg extended and the other leg lifted, perform circular movements with the lifted leg. This exercise is great for improving hip mobility, strengthening the core, and enhancing coordination. Leg Circles help to develop control and balance in the lower body.

Short Box Series

The Short Box Series involves various seated exercises on a box placed on the Reformer. These exercises, including forward flexion, side bending, and twisting, target the core, lower back, and obliques. The Short Box Series enhances core strength, flexibility, and overall torso stability.

Adjusting The Reformer For Different Body Types

To get the most out of Reformer exercises, it's crucial to adjust the equipment according to individual body types and needs. Here's how you can make these adjustments:

Spring Tension

The Reformer has adjustable springs that provide resistance. For beginners or those with less strength, lighter springs are preferable. As strength improves, you can gradually increase the spring tension to challenge yourself further. Proper adjustment ensures the exercises are performed effectively and safely.

Football Position

The footbar can be moved to accommodate different leg lengths and exercise requirements. Adjusting the footbar height ensures proper alignment and comfort during footwork and other leg exercises. Make sure it's set at a level that allows for a full range of motion without straining.

Carriage Placement

The carriage can be adjusted to suit the length of your body. Positioning the carriage correctly helps maintain proper alignment and balance during exercises. Ensure it's set so that you can perform movements smoothly and without unnecessary strain.

Headrest and Shoulder Blocks

The headrest and shoulder blocks can be adjusted to support different body sizes and to ensure proper alignment. Proper placement of these components prevents discomfort and supports effective exercise execution.

Safety And Maintenance Of The Reformer

Regular Inspections

Inspect the Reformer regularly to ensure that all parts are in good working condition. Check for any wear and tear on springs, straps, and the carriage. Address any issues promptly to avoid accidents or equipment failure during workouts.

Cleaning

Keep the Reformer clean by wiping down surfaces after each use. Use appropriate cleaning solutions that do not damage the equipment. Regular cleaning prevents the buildup of sweat and dirt, maintaining a hygienic and pleasant workout environment.

Adjustments and Repairs

Make sure that all adjustments, such as spring tension and football height, are securely set before beginning a workout. If you notice any malfunction or unusual noise during use, consult a professional for repairs. Proper maintenance ensures the Reformer remains safe and effective.

Proper Use

Always follow the recommended guidelines for using the Reformer. Avoid overloading the springs and ensure proper technique to prevent injury. Educate yourself on the correct use of the equipment and adhere to safety protocols during exercises.

Integrating Reformer Workouts Into Your Routine

Consistency

Incorporate Reformer workouts into your weekly fitness routine to achieve the best results.

Aim for at least two to three sessions per week, gradually increasing the frequency as your body adapts. Consistent practice will help you build strength, flexibility, and overall fitness.

Combining with Other Exercises

Integrate Reformer exercises with other forms of physical activity, such as cardio or strength training, for a well-rounded fitness regimen.

Combining different types of exercises enhances overall fitness and prevents workout monotony.

Setting Goals

Establish clear fitness goals and tailor your Reformer workouts to achieve them. Whether you're focusing on strength, flexibility, or injury rehabilitation, customizing your sessions based on your goals will lead to more effective and satisfying results.

Tracking Progress

Keep track of your progress by recording your workouts and noting any improvements in strength, flexibility, or endurance.

Regularly reviewing your progress will help you stay motivated and adjust your routine as needed to continue challenging yourself.

Seeking Professional Guidance

Consider working with a certified Pilates instructor, especially if you're new to Reformer exercises. Professional guidance ensures that you perform exercises correctly and safely, maximizing the benefits and minimizing the risk of injury.

CHAPTER SIX

PILATES FOR SPECIFIC CONDITIONS

Pilates For Back Pain Relief

Pilates is a gentle yet effective exercise method that can significantly alleviate back pain. The core principles of Pilates—stability, strength, and flexibility—make it an ideal choice for those suffering from back discomfort. By focusing on exercises that strengthen the core muscles, Pilates helps support the spine and improve posture, which can reduce strain on the back.

One of the foundational exercises for back pain relief is the "Pelvic Curl." This move strengthens the lower back and glutes while improving spinal flexibility. Begin by lying on your back with your knees bent and feet flat on the floor. Slowly lift your hips towards the ceiling, articulating your spine one vertebra at a time. Hold for a few seconds before gently rolling back down.

This exercise helps to align the spine and relieve tension in the lower back.

Another beneficial exercise is the "Single Leg Stretch," which targets the abdominal muscles and helps stabilize the pelvis.

Lie on your back, bring one knee towards your chest while extending the opposite leg, and switch legs in a controlled manner. This exercise improves core strength and helps support the back during daily activities.

Pilates For Joint Health And Mobility

Pilates can enhance joint health and mobility by improving the strength and flexibility of the muscles surrounding the joints. This approach helps to maintain or increase the range of motion and reduce stiffness.

For joint health, exercises like the "Shoulder Bridge" are highly effective. Lie on your back with knees bent and feet hip-width apart.

Lift your hips towards the ceiling while pressing your shoulders into the mat. This exercise strengthens the glutes and lower back while improving flexibility in the hips and spine.

The "Saw" exercise is another excellent choice for joint mobility. Sit with your legs extended in front of you and your feet flexed.

Extend your arms to the sides and twist your torso to reach one hand towards the opposite foot, mimicking a sawing motion.

This exercise increases spinal mobility and stretches the hamstrings, enhancing overall joint function.

Pilates For Post-Surgery Recovery

Post-surgery recovery can benefit greatly from Pilates, as it focuses on gradual strengthening and flexibility exercises that promote healing without undue stress on the body. Pilates helps rebuild strength and function in a controlled and supportive manner.

After surgery, start with gentle exercises like the "Arm Circles" to regain shoulder mobility. Stand or sit with arms extended to the sides, and make small circles with your hands. This exercise improves shoulder joint movement and helps reduce stiffness.

The "Leg Slides" exercise is beneficial for lower body recovery. Lie on your back with your knees bent and feet flat on the floor. Slowly slide one leg out straight while keeping the foot on the floor, then return to the starting position. This exercise strengthens the core and improves lower body mobility, essential for recovery.

Modifications For Chronic Conditions

For individuals with chronic conditions, Pilates exercises can be modified to accommodate specific needs while still providing therapeutic benefits. It's important to work with a trained Pilates instructor who can tailor exercises to individual limitations and capabilities.

For those with arthritis, modifications like using a chair for support during exercises can be helpful. Exercises such as seated marches or seated leg lifts can help maintain joint mobility and reduce pain without putting excess pressure on the joints.

In cases of fibromyalgia, exercises should be performed at a slower pace and with minimal resistance. The "Cat-Cow Stretch," which involves gently arching and rounding the back while on hands and knees, can help alleviate stiffness and improve flexibility.

Real-Life Success Stories And Testimonials

Hearing from individuals who have experienced success with Pilates for therapy can be inspiring and motivating. Many people have found relief and improved their quality of life through Pilates.

For example, Jane, a 52-year-old with chronic back pain, found significant relief through a consistent Pilates practice. She started with basic exercises and gradually incorporated more challenging movements. Jane's story highlights how Pilates can be a transformative tool for managing chronic pain and improving overall well-being.

Another success story comes from Tom, who underwent knee surgery and used Pilates to aid his recovery. By following a modified Pilates routine, Tom was able to regain strength and mobility in his knee, allowing him to return to his active lifestyle much sooner than anticipated. His experience underscores the effectiveness of Pilates in post-surgery rehabilitation.

These real-life examples illustrate the practical benefits of Pilates in managing specific conditions and offer hope to those seeking relief through this therapeutic exercise method.

CHAPTER SEVEN

ADVANCED PILATES TECHNIQUES

Transitioning From Beginner To Advanced Exercises

Transitioning from beginner to advanced Pilates exercises involves gradually increasing the complexity and intensity of your workouts. Start by mastering foundational moves like the Hundred and Roll-Up, ensuring proper form and core engagement. As you gain confidence, incorporate more challenging exercises such as the Teaser or the Advanced Plank, which demand greater balance and strength.

A key aspect of this progression is understanding how to listen to your body. Pay attention to signals of fatigue or strain, and adjust your routine accordingly. It's also beneficial to work with a certified Pilates instructor who can guide you through advanced techniques and ensure you're performing exercises correctly to avoid injuries.

Challenging The Body With Complex Movements

Advanced Pilates techniques often involve complex movements that challenge your body in new ways. Exercises such as the Leg Circles and the Scissors require precise control and coordination. These movements engage multiple muscle groups simultaneously, enhancing overall strength and flexibility.

To perform these exercises effectively, focus on maintaining proper alignment and controlled breathing. This not only maximizes the benefits but also helps in preventing injuries. Incorporating movements like the Snake or the Swan Dive can also push your limits, providing a full-body workout that improves endurance and stability.

Using Advanced Equipment: Cadillac, Chair, And Barrel

Advanced Pilates equipment, including the Cadillac, Chair, and Barrel, offers a wide range of exercises that can further enhance your practice. The Cadillac, with its adjustable springs and bars, allows for dynamic stretching and strengthening exercises. For example, the Cadillac can be used for exercises like the Roll Down or the Pull-Up to challenge your core and improve flexibility.

The Pilates Chair, on the other hand, provides resistance training that targets smaller stabilizing muscles. Exercises such as the Leg Press or the Short Box Series on the Chair can intensify your workout and improve your overall strength.

The Barrel, with its curved surface, is excellent for deep stretching and spinal articulation. Using the Barrel for exercises like the Back Stretch or the Side Sit-Up can enhance your flexibility and core strength. Familiarity with these pieces of equipment will help you perform advanced Pilates techniques with greater precision and effectiveness.

Combining Pilates With Other Fitness Routines

Integrating Pilates with other fitness routines can create a balanced workout regimen that addresses various aspects of fitness. For instance, combining Pilates with strength training can improve muscle tone and endurance. Pilates exercises complement weight lifting by enhancing core stability and flexibility.

Incorporating Pilates into a cardio routine can also be beneficial. Performing Pilates exercises before or after a cardio session can enhance muscle activation and recovery. Additionally, adding Pilates to activities like running or cycling can help in improving posture, alignment, and overall performance.

When combining Pilates with other fitness routines, it's crucial to maintain a balanced approach. Ensure that you allocate time for recovery and adjust the intensity of each workout to prevent overtraining and reduce the risk of injury.

Preventing Injuries During Advanced Practice

Preventing injuries during advanced Pilates practice involves several key strategies. First, always prioritize proper technique over the number of repetitions or the intensity of the exercises. Incorrect form can lead to strain or injury, especially when performing complex movements.

Warm up thoroughly before starting your routine. A proper warm-up prepares your muscles and joints for the workout, reducing the risk of injuries. Include dynamic stretches and low-intensity movements to increase blood flow and flexibility.

Incorporate cooldown and stretching exercises at the end of your session to promote recovery and maintain flexibility. Pay attention to any signs of discomfort or pain, and modify exercises as needed. Regularly consulting with a Pilates instructor can provide additional guidance on form and technique, ensuring a safe and effective practice.

CHAPTER EIGHT

CREATING A PERSONALIZED PILATES PROGRAM

Assessing Individual Needs And Goals

When embarking on a Pilates journey, the first step is to assess your individual needs and goals. This process begins with a self-evaluation or a consultation with a qualified Pilates instructor.

Identify any specific physical conditions, such as chronic pain, injuries, or areas of stiffness. Understand your fitness level, from beginner to advanced, to tailor your program accordingly. Setting clear, achievable goals is crucial—whether you aim to improve flexibility, strengthen core muscles, enhance posture, or relieve stress.

By understanding your starting point and desired outcomes, you can create a personalized program that meets your unique requirements.

Designing A Balanced Weekly Pilates Schedule

A balanced weekly Pilates schedule is key to ensuring comprehensive body conditioning and preventing overuse injuries. Start by allocating time for Pilates sessions at least three to four times a week.

Mix in different types of workouts to target various muscle groups and maintain overall balance.

For example, alternate between core-focused sessions, full-body workouts, and flexibility routines. Incorporate rest days or lighter sessions to allow for muscle recovery. This balanced approach not only maximizes the benefits of Pilates but also keeps your routine interesting and sustainable over the long term.

Mixing Mat And Equipment Workouts

To keep your Pilates routine dynamic and effective, mix mat and equipment workouts. Mat exercises primarily use your body weight for resistance and focus on fundamental movements that build strength, flexibility, and control.

Equipment workouts, such as those using the Reformer, Cadillac, or Wunda Chair, add resistance and variety, challenging your muscles in new ways. Incorporating both types of workouts ensures a well-rounded program. For instance, you might start the week with a mat session to engage your core, follow with a Reformer class for resistance training, and end with a Cadillac session to enhance flexibility and balance.

Adapting Routines For Progress And Variety

As you advance in your Pilates practice, it's essential to adapt routines to match your progress and keep your workouts varied. Gradually increase the difficulty of exercises by adding more repetitions, increasing resistance, or incorporating advanced moves.

Introduce new exercises or variations to target different muscle groups and prevent plateaus. Consider trying different class styles or specialty equipment to keep your routine fresh and challenging.

Adapting your Pilates routines not only helps you progress but also maintains your motivation and enjoyment.

Evaluating And Adjusting Your Program Over Time

Regularly evaluating and adjusting your Pilates program ensures it continues to meet your evolving needs and goals. Periodically review your progress by noting improvements in strength, flexibility, and overall well-being. Reflect on any challenges or areas that need additional focus. Based on this evaluation, make necessary adjustments to your schedule, exercise selection, and intensity. Consulting with a Pilates instructor can provide valuable feedback and guidance for fine-tuning your program. By staying attuned to your body and progress, you can continually optimize your Pilates practice for long-term success and satisfaction.

CHAPTER NINE

COMMON CONCERNS AND FAQS

Addressing Common Fears And Misconceptions

Many people considering Pilates for therapy often have concerns or misconceptions about the practice. One common fear is that Pilates might be too difficult or not suitable for beginners. In reality, Pilates is highly adaptable and can be modified to suit individuals of all fitness levels. Whether you're just starting or recovering from an injury, Pilates exercises can be tailored to your specific needs, ensuring a safe and effective practice.

Another misconception is that Pilates is only for people looking to improve flexibility. While flexibility is a benefit, Pilates also focuses on strengthening core muscles, improving posture, and enhancing overall body alignment. It's a comprehensive approach that integrates strength, balance, and coordination.

Some also worry that Pilates requires special equipment or that it is expensive. Many effective Pilates exercises can be performed using just a mat, and there are various online resources and classes available at different price points. It's possible to achieve significant benefits from Pilates without investing in costly equipment or classes.

Dealing With Soreness And Fatigue

Experiencing soreness after starting Pilates is normal, especially if you're new to the practice or have increased the intensity of your workouts. This muscle soreness, often referred to as delayed onset muscle soreness (DOMS), is a sign that your muscles are adapting and strengthening. To alleviate soreness, ensure you're properly warming up before exercise and cooling down afterward. Gentle stretching and hydration can also help reduce muscle tightness.

Fatigue is another aspect to manage, especially if you're incorporating Pilates into a busy routine. It's essential to listen to your body and not push yourself too hard. If you're feeling overly fatigued, it's okay to take a rest day or reduce the intensity of your workouts. Balanced nutrition and adequate rest are crucial for recovery and maintaining energy levels.

Finding The Right Balance Between Effort And Rest

Finding the right balance between effort and rest is key to maximizing the benefits of Pilates and preventing overtraining. Start with a manageable routine and gradually increase the intensity as your strength and endurance build. It's important to include rest days in your schedule to allow your muscles time to recover and grow stronger.

A balanced approach also involves paying attention to how your body feels during and after workouts. If you notice persistent pain or discomfort, it may be a sign that you're pushing yourself too hard. Adjust your routine as needed and consider consulting a Pilates instructor or physical therapist to ensure you're performing exercises correctly and safely.

Answers to Frequently Asked Questions About Pilates

Q: How often should I practice Pilates for therapy?

A: For optimal results, practicing Pilates 2-3 times a week is generally recommended. This frequency allows your muscles to adapt and strengthen them effectively without leading to overuse or burnout. However, individual needs may vary, so it's important to tailor the frequency to your specific goals and fitness level.

Q: Can Pilates help with back pain?

A: Yes, Pilates is often used to help alleviate back pain by strengthening the core muscles that support the spine. It promotes better posture and alignment, which can reduce strain on the back. Always consult with a healthcare provider before starting Pilates for back pain to ensure it's appropriate for your condition.

Q: Do I need a Pilates instructor?

A: While it's possible to practice Pilates on your own, especially with the help of online resources, working with a certified Pilates instructor can be beneficial, particularly if you're new to the practice. An instructor can provide personalized guidance, correct your form, and help you avoid injuries.

Q: Can I do Pilates if I have a specific injury or medical condition?

A: Pilates can often be adapted for various injuries and medical conditions, but it's crucial to consult with your healthcare provider before starting. A qualified Pilates instructor or physical therapist can help tailor exercises to accommodate your condition and ensure a safe practice.

Tips For Staying Committed And Enjoying Your Practice

Staying committed to Pilates involves setting realistic goals and finding enjoyment in your practice. Start by setting small, achievable goals that motivate you and track your progress. Celebrate your successes, no matter how small, to stay encouraged.

Incorporate Pilates into your routine in a way that fits your lifestyle. Whether it's a morning practice, a lunchtime session, or an evening wind-down, finding a time that works best for you will help maintain consistency.

Make your practice enjoyable by varying your workouts. Incorporate different exercises and try new routines to keep things fresh and exciting. Joining a class or practicing with a friend can also add a social element that enhances motivation and enjoyment.

Remember to be patient with yourself. Progress in Pilates, as with any exercise, takes time. Focus on the positive changes in your body and mind, and keep your practice enjoyable and rewarding.

www.ingramcontent.com/pod-product-compliance
Lightning Source LLC
Chambersburg PA
CBHW071840210526
45479CB00001B/214